Weight Loss for Women

Lose Weight Fast Up to 14lbs in Just 1 Week –

The Scientifically Proven Method that Will Help You to Burn Fat, Boost Energy and Eliminate Cravings

Is this the book for you?

Do you **STRUGGLE** to **LOSE WEIGHT?** Or would you like to **LOSE WEIGHT FASTER?** If you've answered **'YES'** to either or both of these questions then **CONGRATULATIONS...! YOU'VE COME TO THE RIGHT PLACE!** The sad truth is that the conventional idea of **'EATING LESS'** and **'EXERCISING MORE'**– doesn't work in the long term. Counting calories, exercising for hours every day and trying to ignore your hunger? That's needless suffering that wastes your precious time & energy and also depletes your willpower. Eventually almost everyone gives up. That's why we have an obesity epidemic! Fortunately there's a better way. **GET READY FOR EFFORTLESS WEIGHT LOSS BECAUSE...EVERYTHING YOU'VE BE TOLD ABOUT WEIGHT LOSS IS WRONG!** It's **NOT** about counting calories... It's **NOT** even about doing more exercise... In fact, the **ANSWER** to **WEIGHT LOSS** is **REALLY VERY SIMPLE...THE BOTTOM LINE?** Your weight is hormonally regulated. All that's needed to ensure **WEIGHT LOSS SUCCESS** is a step by step approach towards reducing your **FAT STORING HORMONE, INSULIN.** This book **OFFERS YOU A SIMPLE PLAN TO HELP YOU DO JUST THAT! SO WHAT ARE YOU WAITING FOR? LET'S JUMP RIGHT IN...**

Legal Disclaimer:

This book contains general information and advice for the reader relating to the potential benefits of adding certain fats to their diet whilst reducing their intake of carbohydrates. It is not intended to replace personalized medical advice. As with any new diet program, the meal plans recommended in this book should be followed only after consulting with your doctor to make sure they are appropriate to your individual circumstances. The author and publisher expressly disclaim responsibility for any adverse effects that may result from the use or application of the information contained within this book.

A Special Acknowledgment to my beautiful children Brandon, Jasmine and Anthony and my Partner Michael for their Love, Support and Patience during the many hours it took to prepare this book.

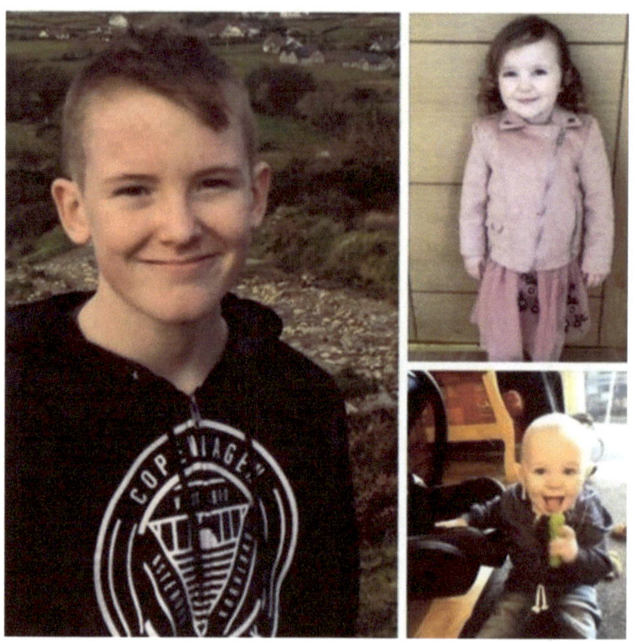

Table of Contents

Introduction

This book was created to help kick start the reader on their weight loss journey. It is designed to help you burn fat, boost energy and eliminate cravings once and for all so that you can lead a healthier, happier, longer life!

Inside this book, you'll find a set of 21 delicious **FAT BURNING RECIPES** that are broken down into 3 meals per day over a 7 day period. Another powerful technique has also been included due to the amazing health benefits that it provides (more on this later).

EACH RECIPE CAN BE PREPARED IN AS LITTLE AS 5 MINUTES making it **IDEAL FOR SOMEONE** looking to lose weight but with **LIMITED TIME TO SPARE** due to a hectic work life/family life schedule.

This is a '**COMPLETE DONE FOR YOU PLAN**' which includes a **BONUS - 1 WEEK SHOPPING LIST& BEAUTIFULLY ILLUSTRATED RECIPE CHARTS THAT CAN BE PRINTED & LAMINATED & PLACED ON YOUR FRIDGE TO OFFER YOU VISUAL GUIDANCE DURING THE 7 DAY PROGRAM**

In total, THERE ARE ONLY 30 INGREDIENTS you will need, making this plan accessible to everyone, even those on a tight budget. Excited? Let's get started...!

Fat Burning Breakfast Day 1

Courgette/Zucchini 75gr

Avocado 60gr (Approx ½ an Avocado)

Feta Cheese 15gr

Eggs x 2

Himalayan Sea Salt (Sprinkle)

Extra Virgin Olive Oil (1tbsp)

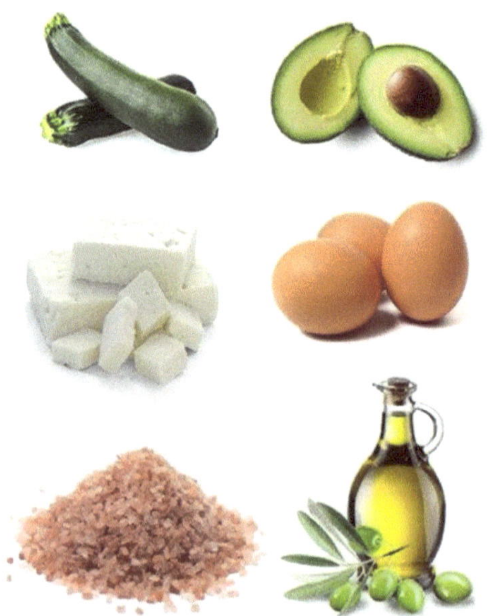

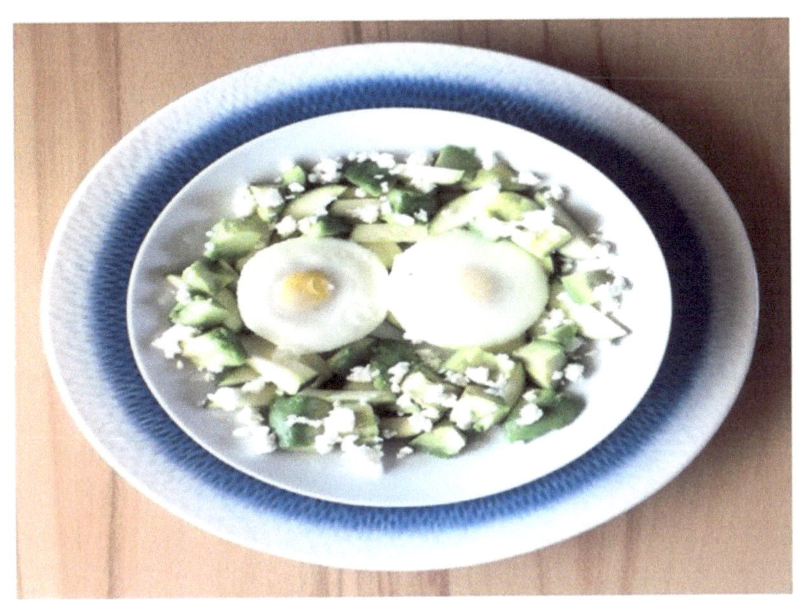

Fat Burning Lunch Day 1

Cauliflower 50gr

Turkey Breast Steak 48gr

Red Onion 15gr

Asparagus x 4 Medium Spears

Himalayan Sea Salt (Sprinkle)

Extra Virgin Olive Oil (2 ¼ tbsp)

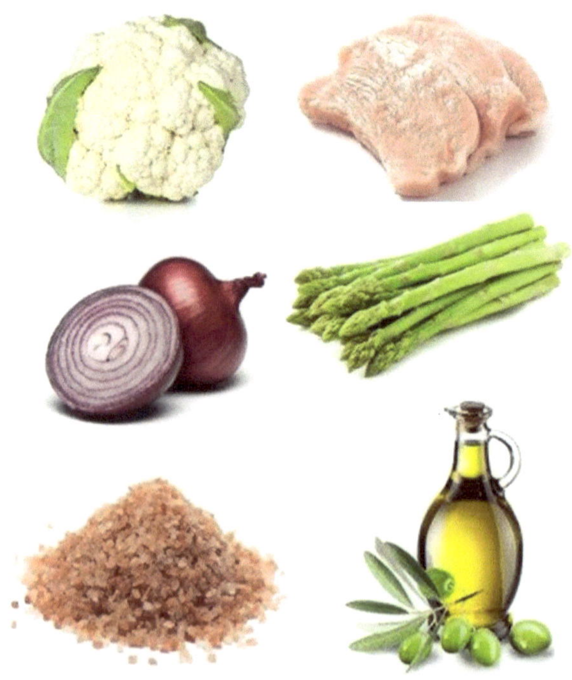

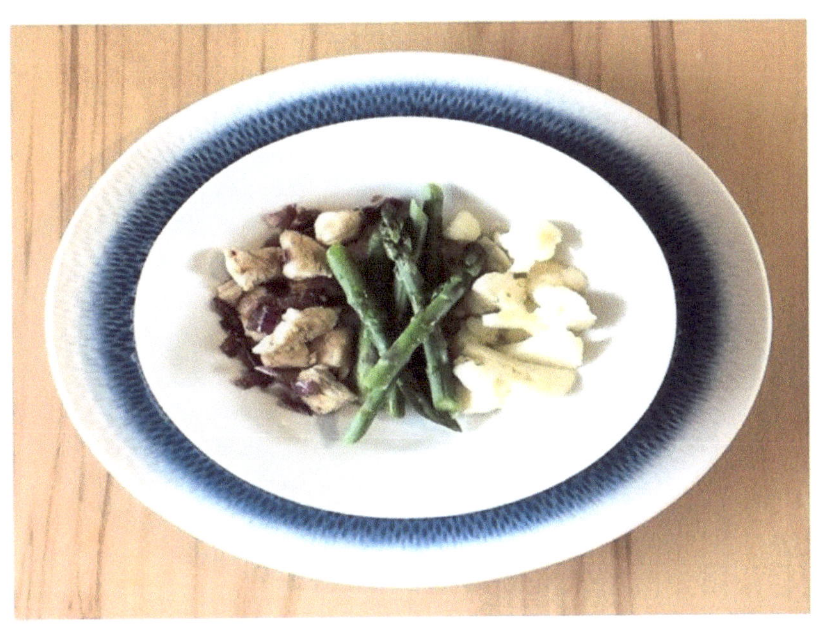

Fat Burning Dinner Day 1

Brussels Sprouts 60gr

Smoked Salmon 45gr

Garlic x 1 Clove

Himalayan Sea Salt (Sprinkle)

Extra Virgin Olive Oil (1 ¾ tbsp)

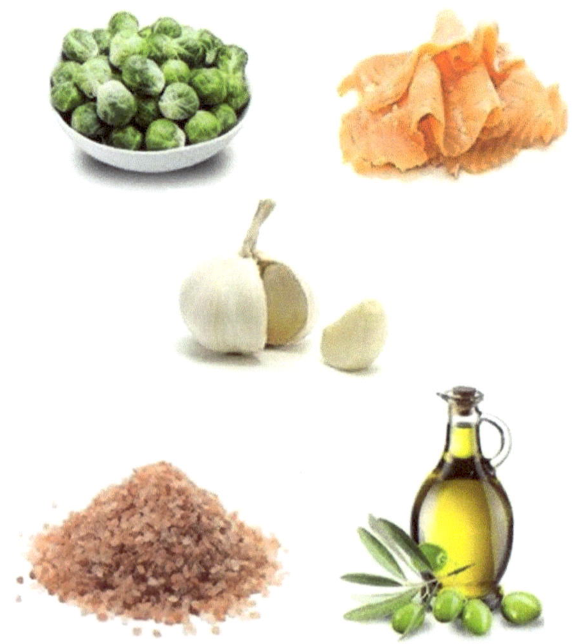

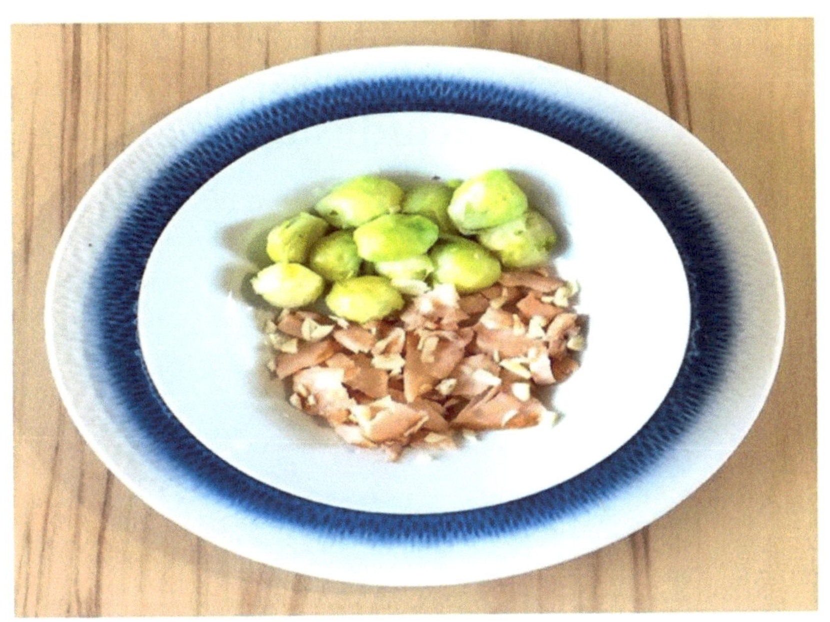

Fat Burning Breakfast Day 2

Dairy Free - (Includes Eggs, Fish & Poultry)

Trout Fillets 62gr

Broccoli 35gr

Butternut Squash 25gr

Asparagus x 2 Medium Spears

Himalayan Sea Salt (Sprinkle)

Extra Virgin Olive Oil (2 ¼ tbsp)

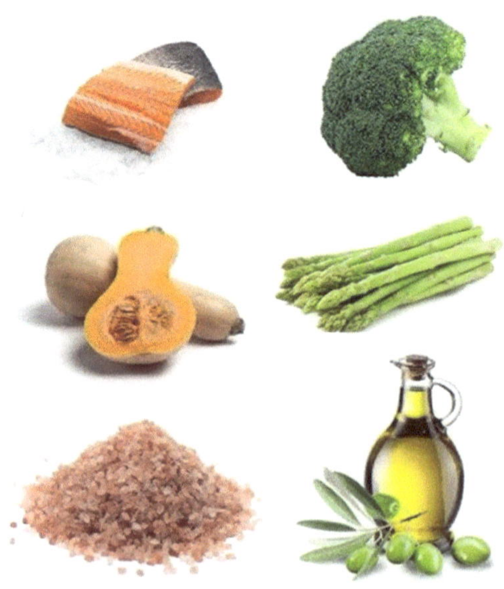

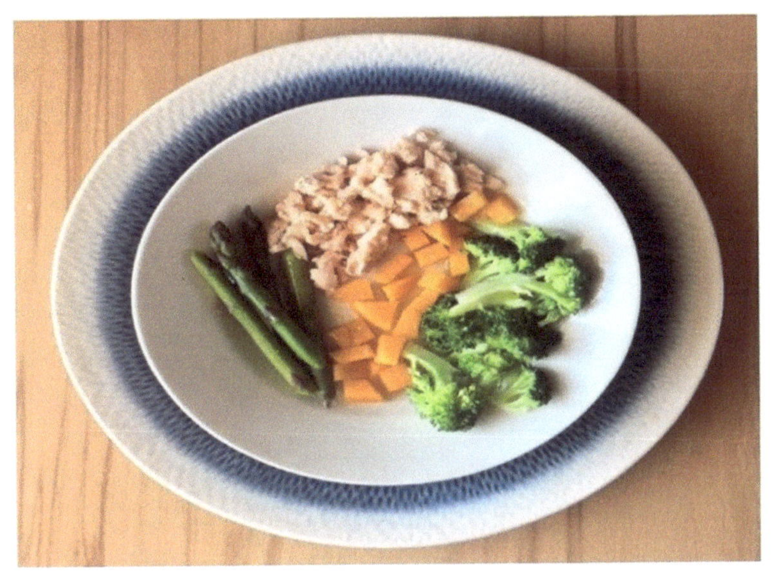

Fat Burning Lunch Day 2

Avocado 60gr - (Approx ½ an Avocado)

Spinach 60gr

Eggs x 2

Garlic x 1 Clove

Himalayan Sea Salt (Sprinkle)

Extra Virgin Olive Oil (1 tbsp)

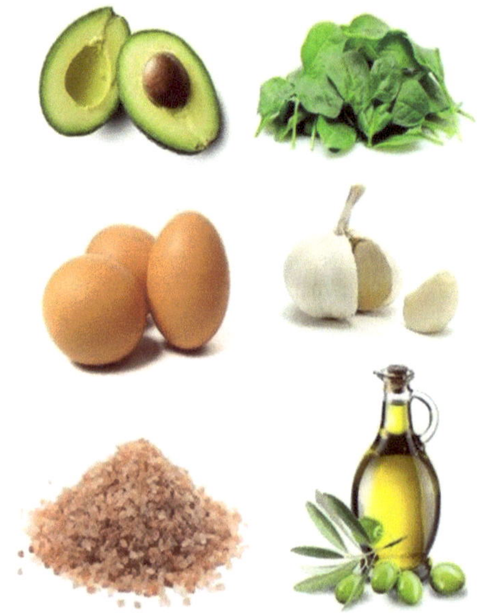

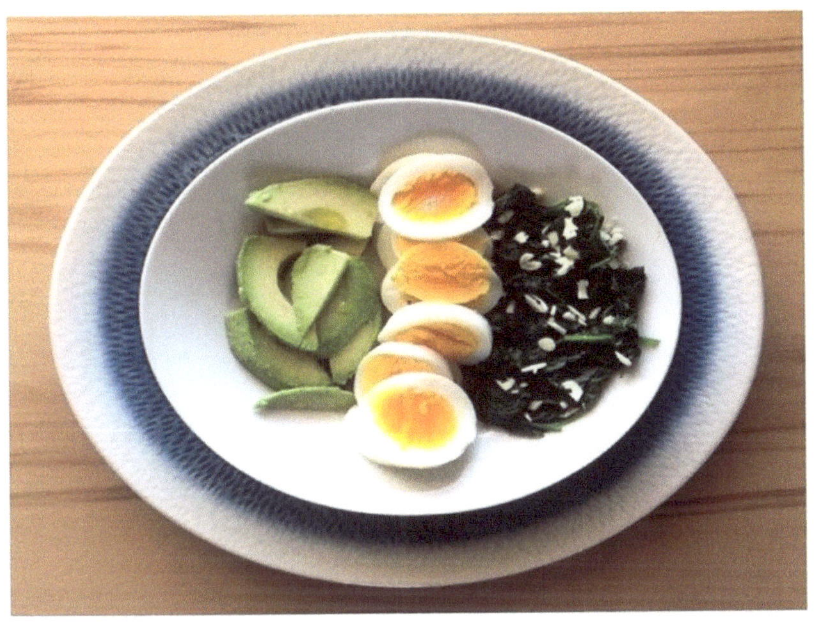

Fat Burning Dinner Day 2

Courgette/Zucchini 75gr

Cooked Chicken Slices 55gr

Cauliflower 50gr

Himalayan Sea Salt (Sprinkle)

Extra Virgin Olive Oil (2tbsp)

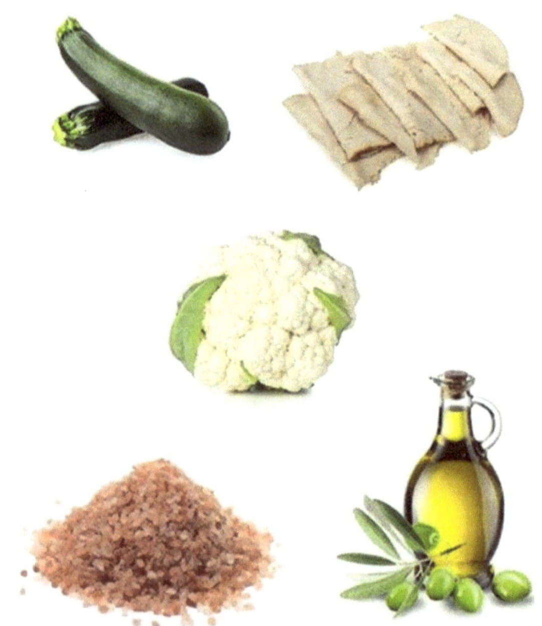

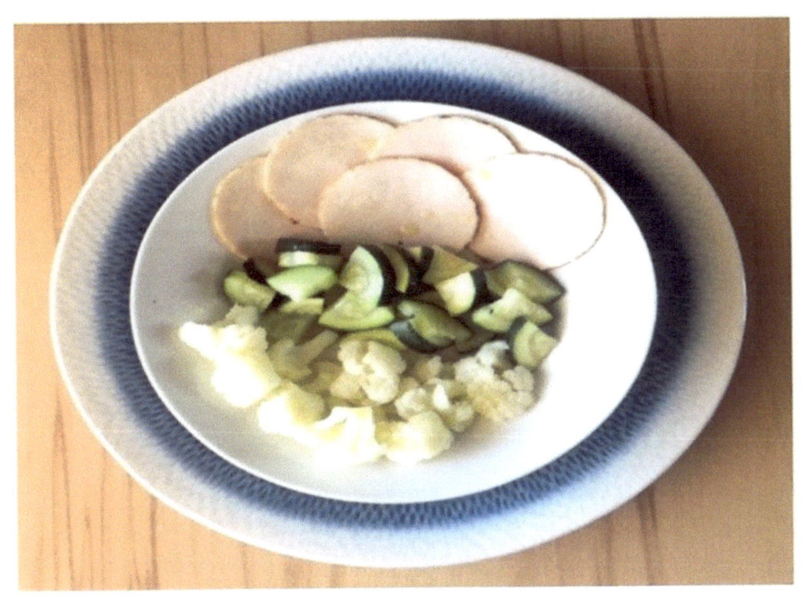

Fat Burning Breakfast Day 3

Fish Free - (Includes Dairy, Eggs & Poultry)

Eggs x 2

Asparagus x 4 Medium Spears

Feta Cheese 15gr

Red Onion 15gr

Himalayan Sea Salt (Sprinkle)

Extra Virgin Olive Oil (1 2/3 tbsp)

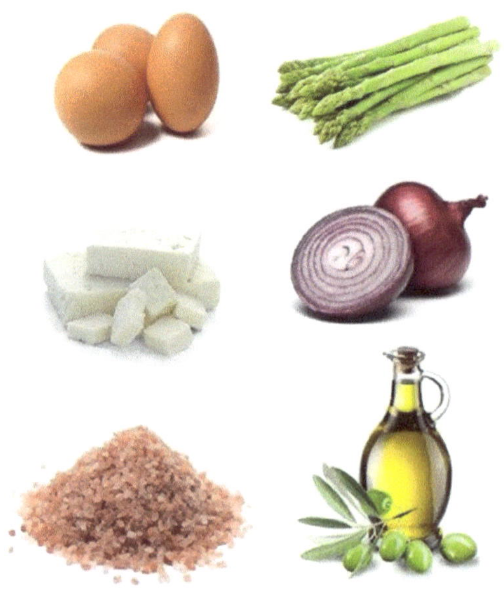

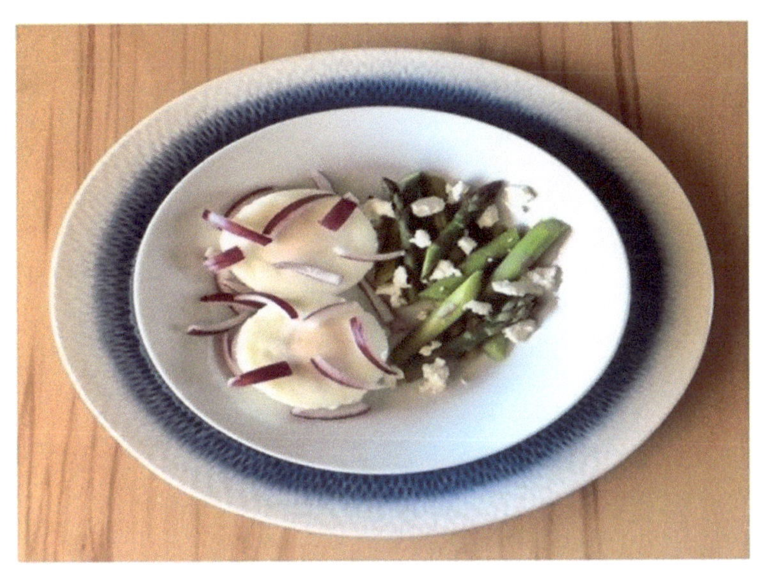

Fat Burning Lunch Day 3

Turkey Breast Steak 48gr

Broccoli 48gr

Pak Choi 40gr

Garlic x 1 Clove

Himalayan Sea Salt (Sprinkle)

Extra Virgin Olive Oil (2tbsp)

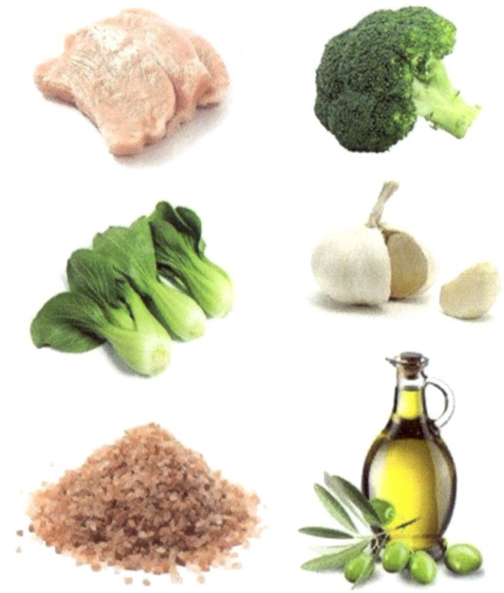

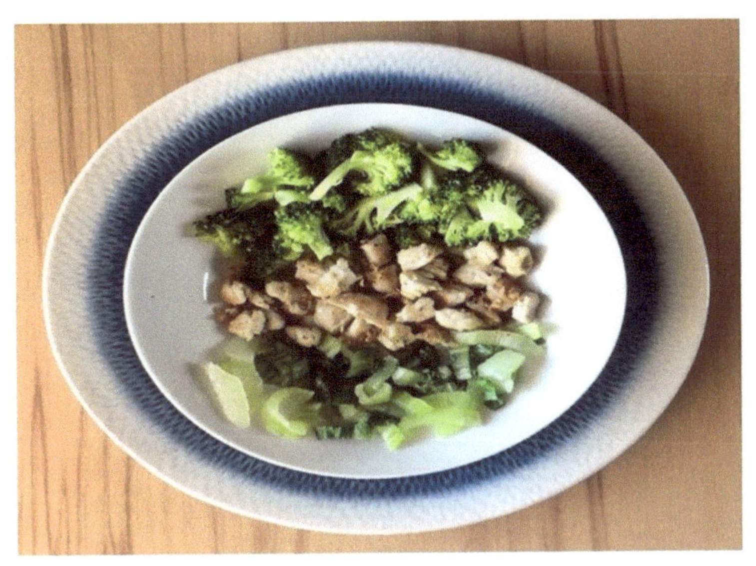

Fat Burning Dinner Day 3

Courgette/Zucchini 75gr

Avocado 60gr - (Approx ½ an Avocado)

Halloumi 45gr

Cauliflower 30gr

Himalayan Sea Salt (Sprinkle)

Extra Virgin Olive Oil (3/4 tbsp)

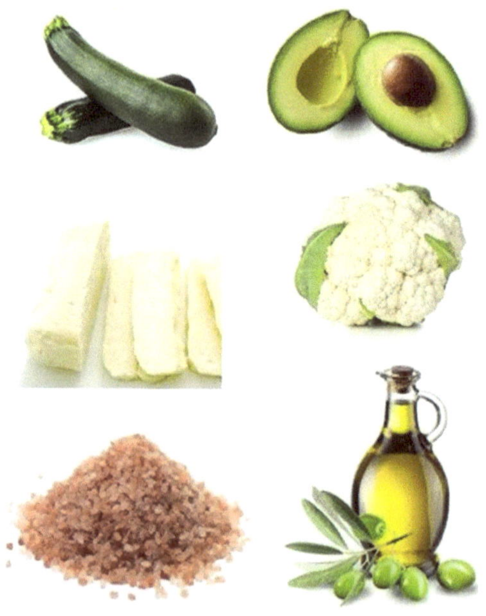

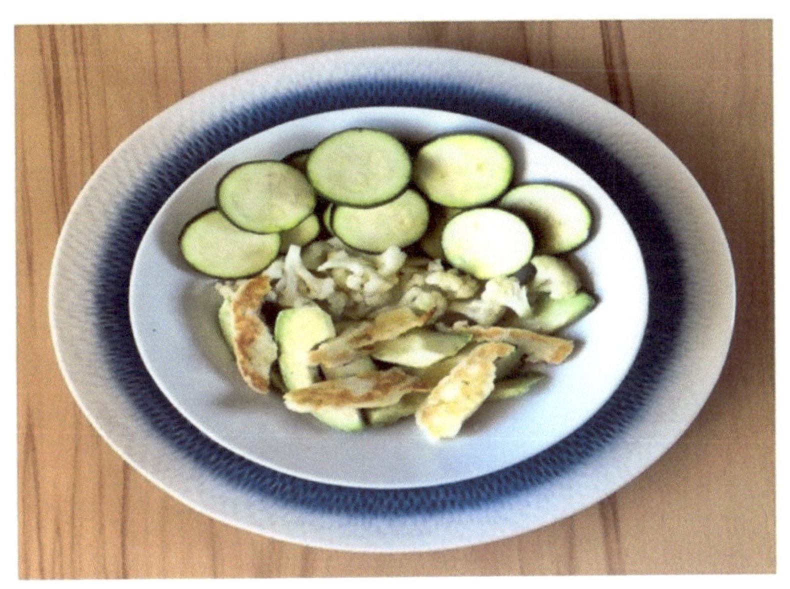

Fat Burning Breakfast Day 4

Avocado 60gr - (Approx ½ an Avocado)

Spinach 60gr

Feta Cheese 15gr

Eggs x 2

Garlic x 1 Clove

Himalayan Sea Salt (Sprinkle)

Extra Virgin Olive Oil (1 tbsp)

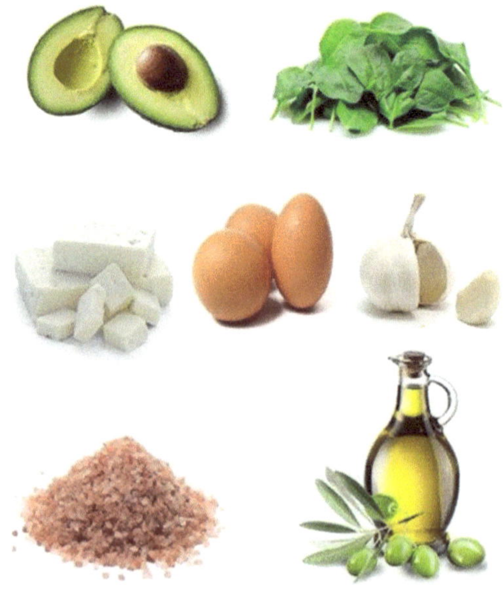

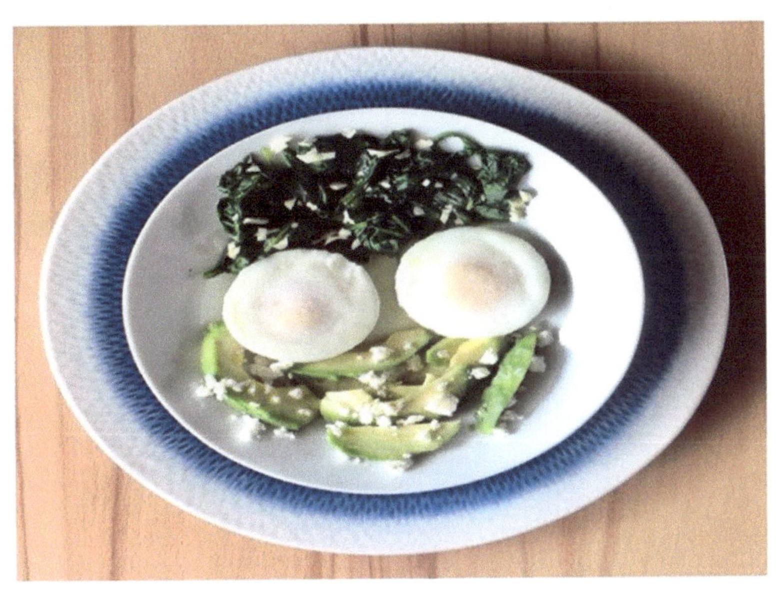

Fat Burning Lunch Day 4

Courgette/Zucchini 75gr

Smoked Salmon 50gr

Cauliflower 30gr

Red Onion 15gr

Himalayan Sea Salt (Sprinkle)

Extra Virgin Olive Oil (2tbsp)

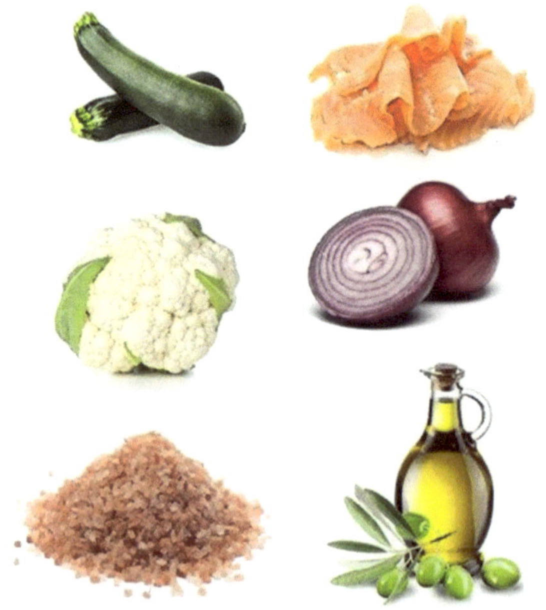

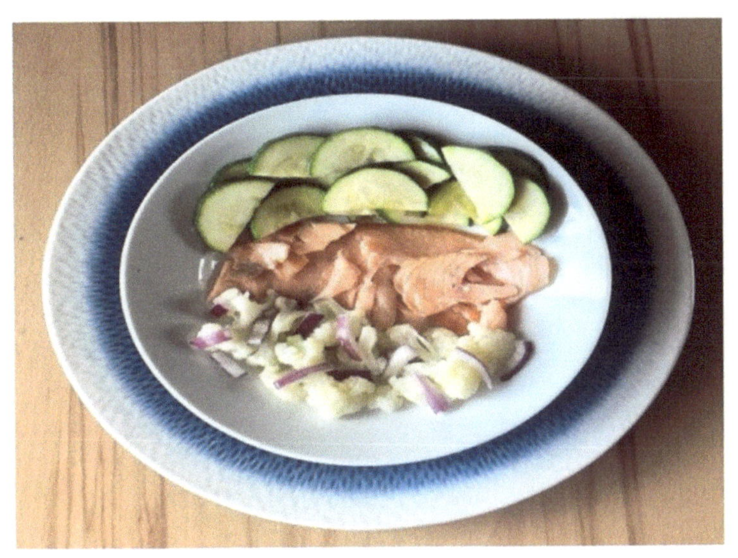

Fat Burning Dinner Day 4

Cooked Chicken Slices 55gr

Broccoli 45gr

Asparagus x 4 Medium Spears

Himalayan Sea Salt (Sprinkle)

Extra Virgin Olive Oil (2tbsp)

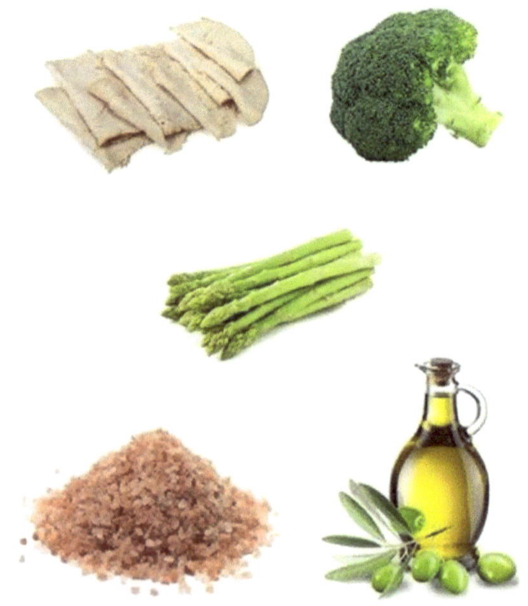

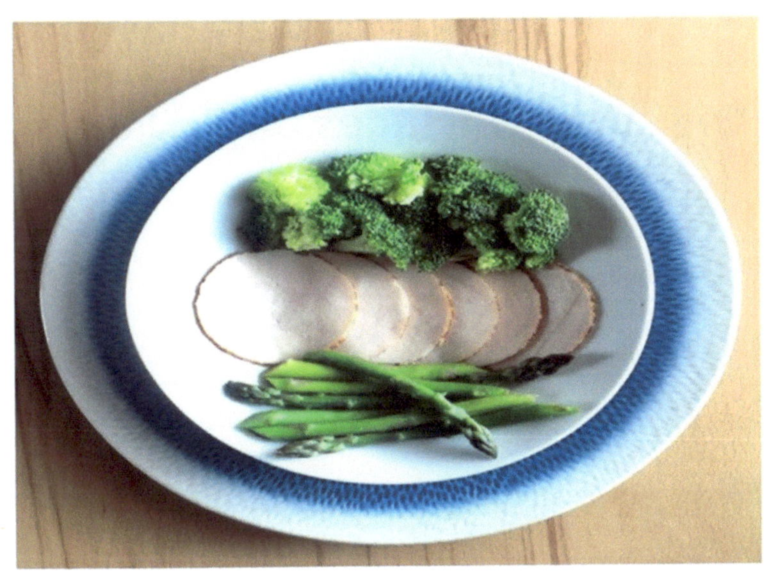

Fat Burning Breakfast Day 5

Egg Free - (Includes Dairy, Fish & Poultry)

Trout Fillets 48gr

Cauliflower 42gr

Pak Choi 25gr

Asparagus x 4 Medium Spears

Himalayan Sea Salt (Sprinkle)

Extra Virgin Olive Oil (2tbsp)

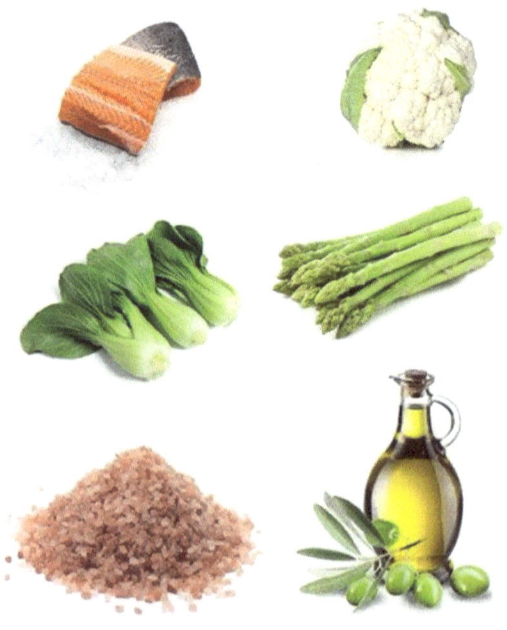

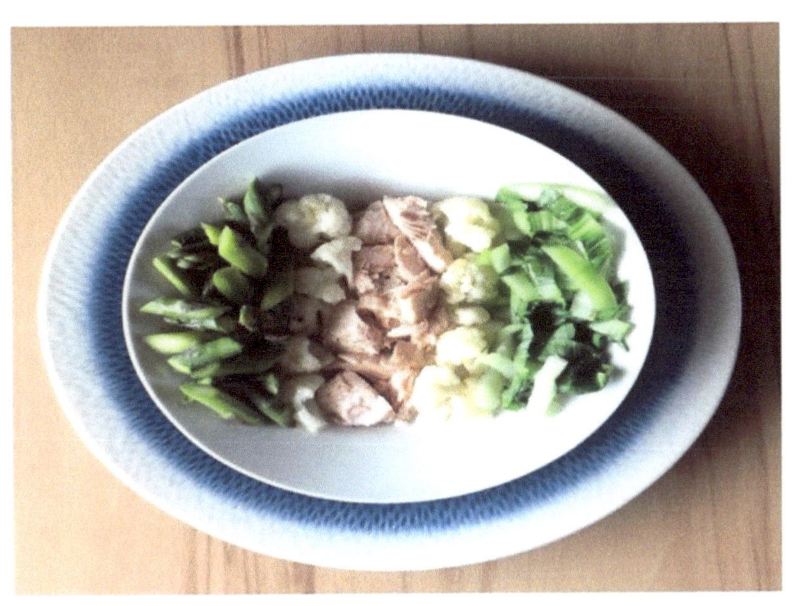

Fat Burning Lunch Day 5

Avocado 60gr - (Approx ½ an Avocado)

Courgette/Zucchini 50gr

Cooked Chicken Slices 35gr

Red Onion 15gr

Feta Cheese 15gr

Himalayan Sea Salt (Sprinkle)

Extra Virgin Olive Oil (3/4 tbsp)

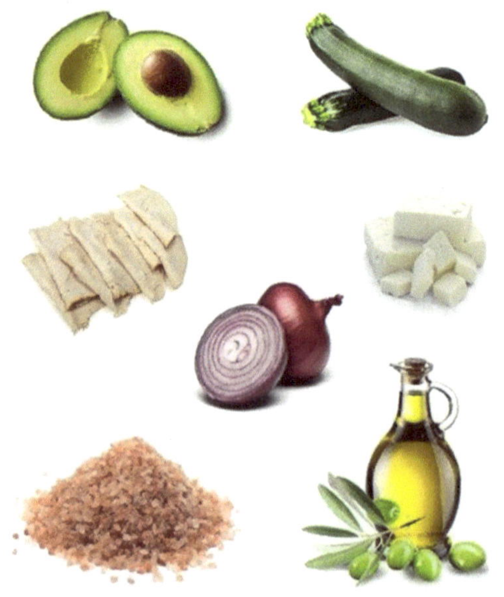

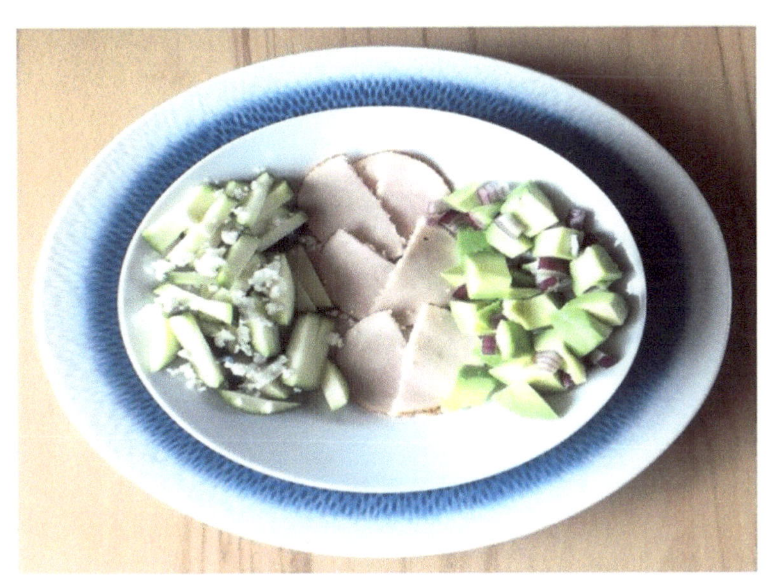

Fat Burning Dinner Day 5

Brussels Sprouts 60gr

Turkey Breast Steak 40gr

Broccoli 32gr

Garlic x 1 Clove

Himalayan Sea Salt (Sprinkle)

Extra Virgin Olive Oil (2tbsp)

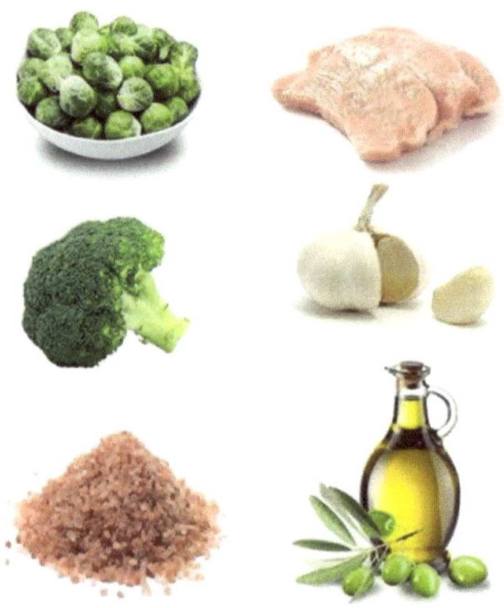

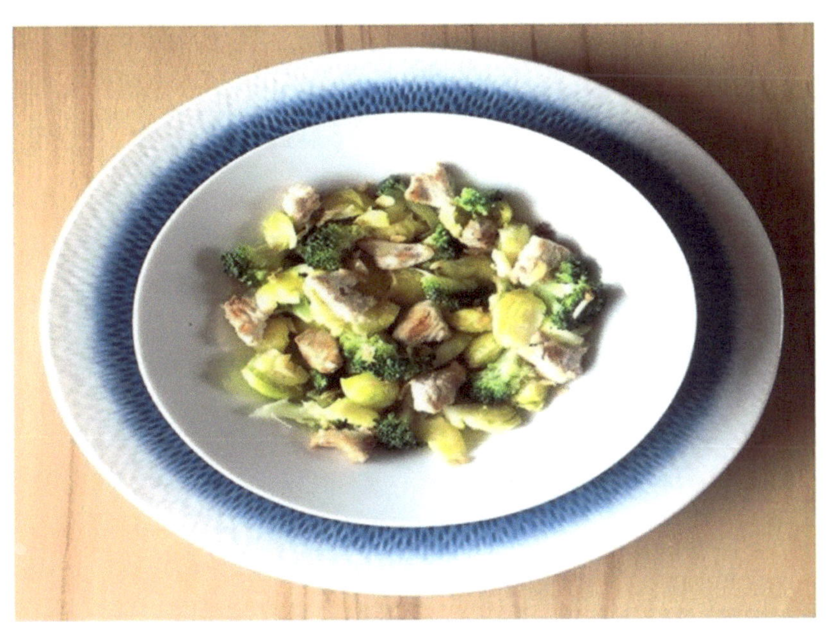

Fat Burning Breakfast Day 6

Dairy & Poultry Free - (Includes Eggs & Fish)

Avocado 50gr

Spinach 50gr

Eggs x 2

Garlic x 1 Clove

Himalayan Sea Salt (Sprinkle)

Extra Virgin Olive Oil (1tbsp)

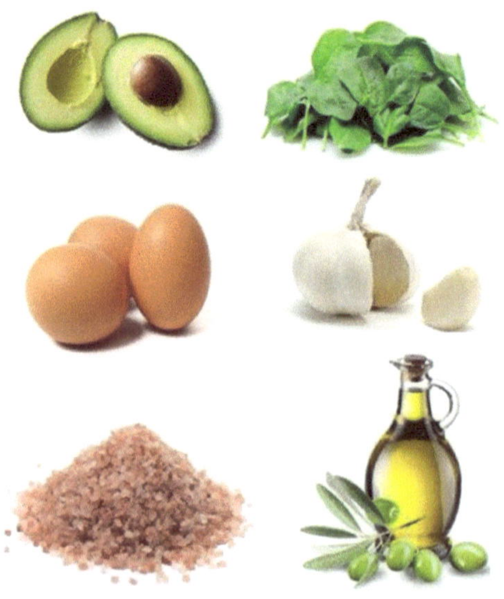

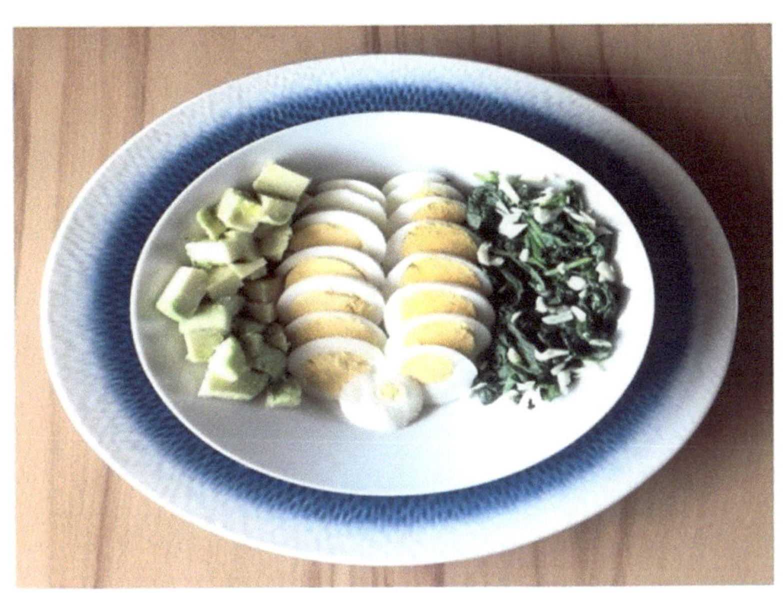

Fat Burning Lunch Day 6

Brussels Sprouts 60gr

Trout Fillet 50gr

Broccoli 50gr

Himalayan Sea Salt (Sprinkle)

Extra Virgin Olive Oil (2tbsp)

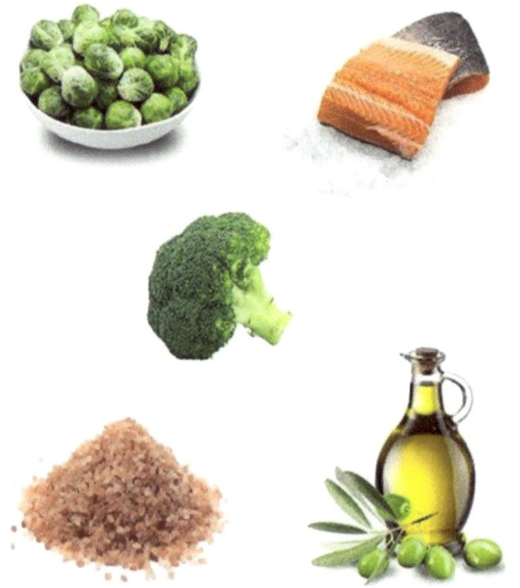

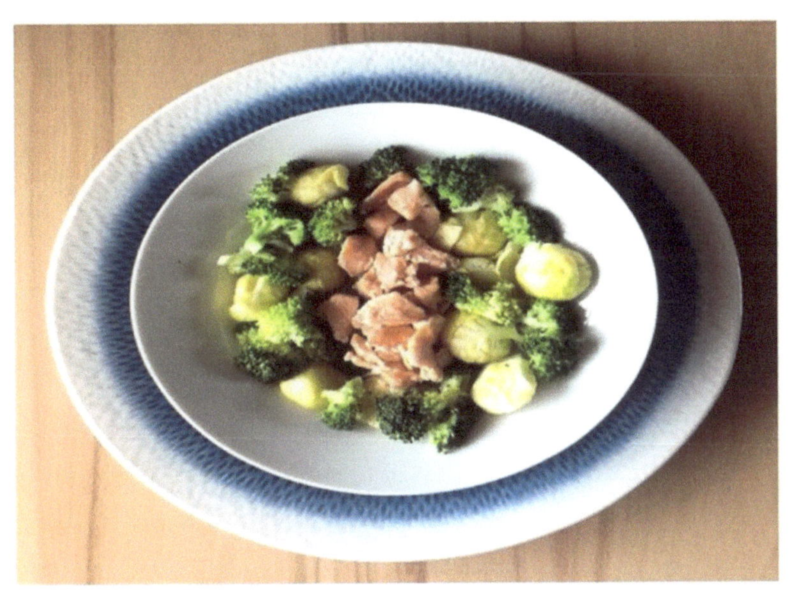

Fat Burning Dinner Day 6

Cauliflower 50gr

Smoked Salmon 46gr

Asparagus x 4 Medium Spears

Himalayan Sea Salt (Sprinkle)

Extra Virgin Olive Oil (2 1/4 tbsp)

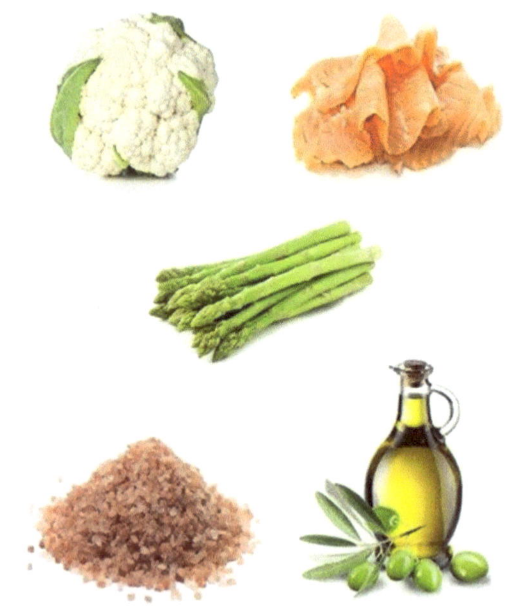

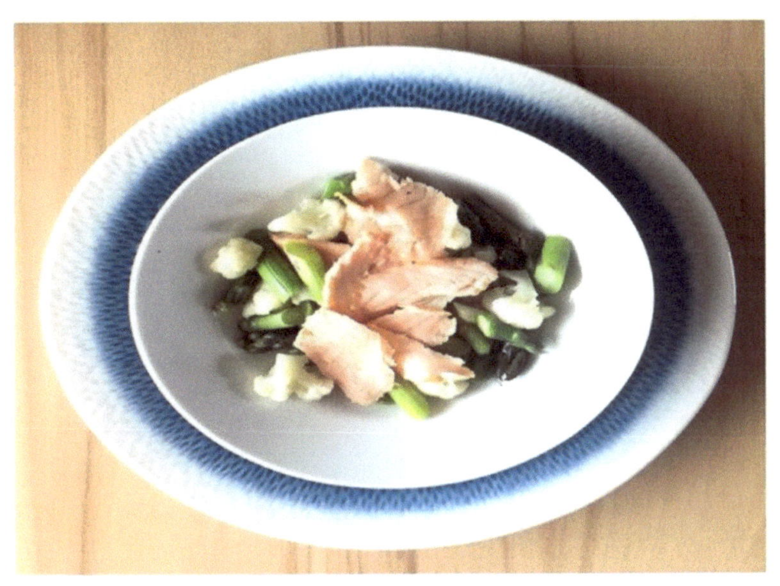

Fat Burning Breakfast Day 7

Dairy, Egg, Fish & Poultry Free

(Includes Nuts & Seeds)

Toasted Pumpkin Seeds 80gr

Courgette/Zucchini 65gr

Pak Choi 25gr

Toasted Flaked Almonds 20gr

Himalayan Sea Salt (Sprinkle)

Extra Virgin Olive Oil (¾ tbsp)

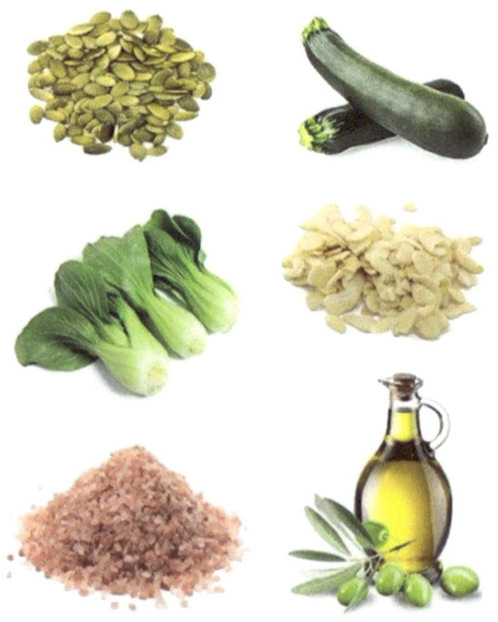

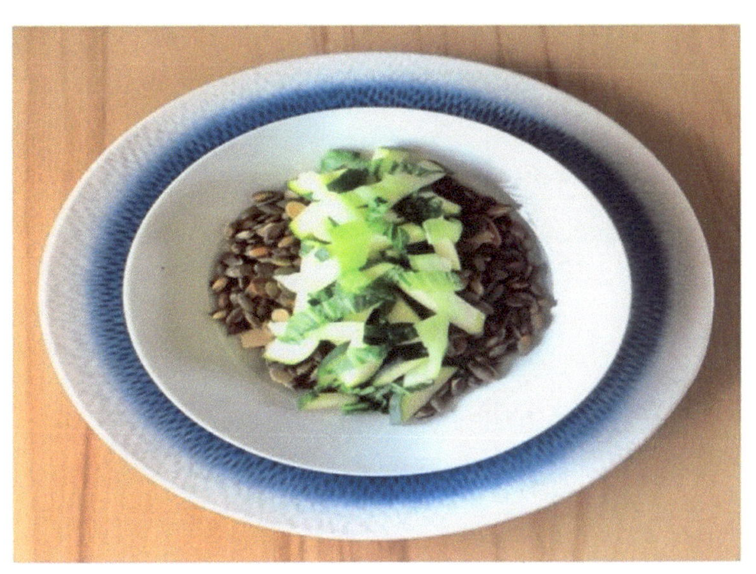

Fat Burning Lunch Day 7

Avocado 45gr

Cauliflower 30gr

Ground Flaxseed 16gr

Pecan Nuts 3gr

Himalayan Sea Salt (Sprinkle)

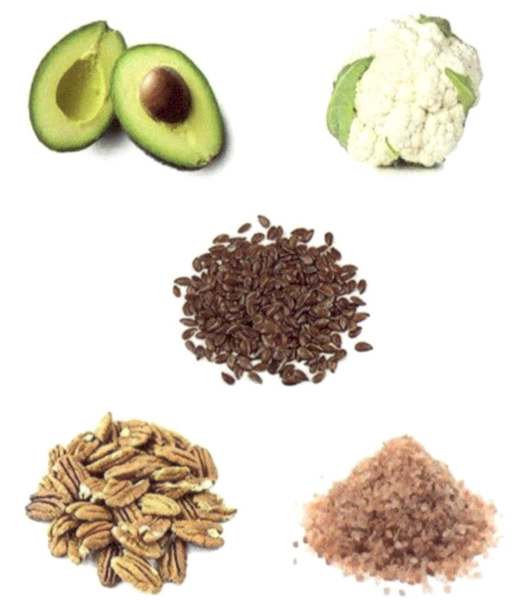

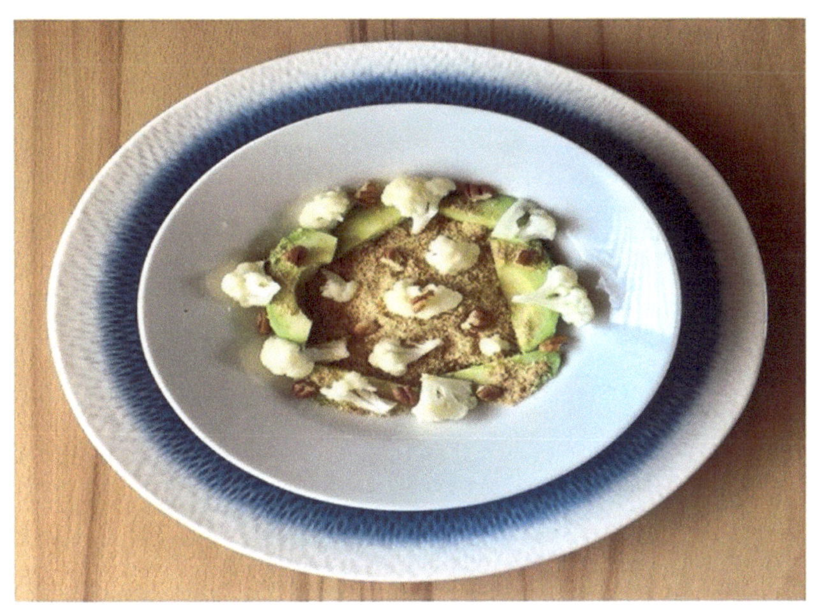

Fat Burning Dinner Day 7

Spinach 55gr

Broccoli 32gr

Macadamia Nuts 10gr

Red Onions 5gr

Walnuts 3gr

Himalayan Sea Salt (Sprinkle)

Extra Virgin Olive Oil (1/3 tbsp)

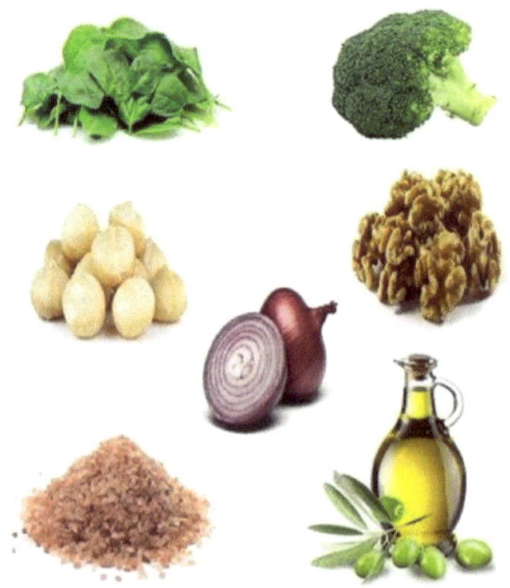

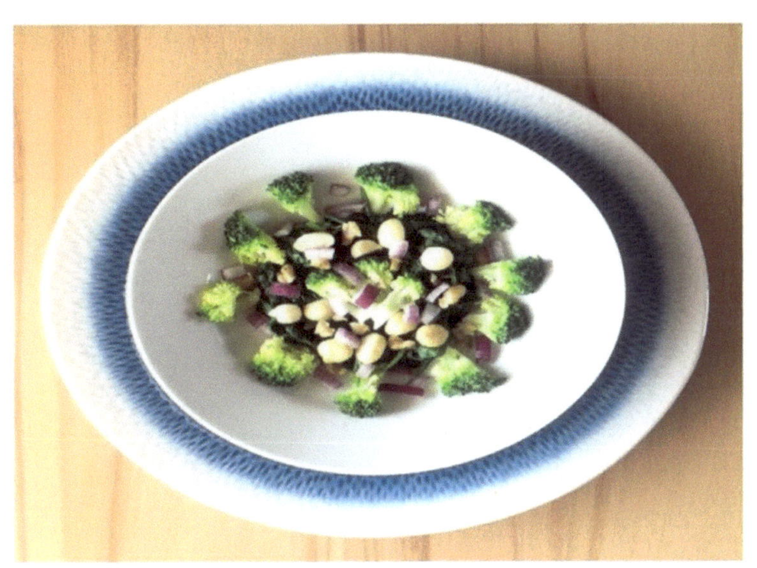

Detox Water Recipe

To make a full pitcher you will need:

1 large cucumber, sliced

1 lime, sliced

1 handful fresh mint leaves

2 quarts water

Method:

Put the cucumber, lime and mint into a large pitcher. Pour water over it and leave to infuse for 2 – 4 hours or overnight

Enjoy!

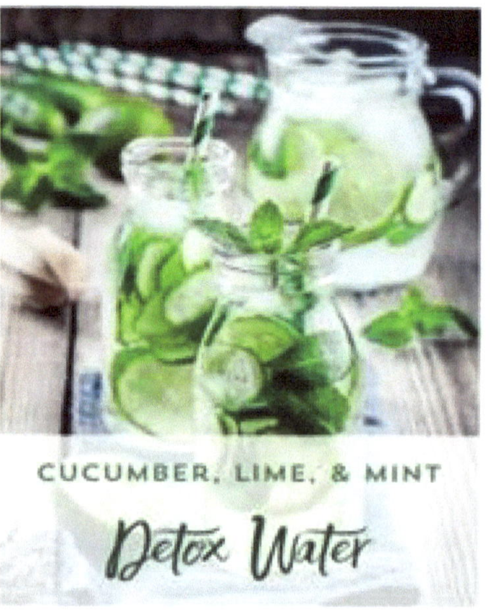

Food Preparation

The following foods can be eaten raw:

Courgette/Zucchini

Walnuts

Avocado

Asparagus

Spinach

Cucumber

Red Onion

Feta Cheese

Flaxseed Milled

Pumpkin Seeds

Almond Flakes

Pecan Nuts

Macadamia Nuts

Garlic

Extra Virgin Olive Oil

Himalayan Sea Salt

The following foods can be gently steamed:

Brussels Sprouts

Pak Choi

Butternut Squash

Trout Fillets

Cauliflower

Broccoli

The following foods can be bought and eaten as they are:

Cooked Chicken Slices

Smoked Salmon

The following foods can be fried:

Turkey Breast Steaks – Cut up in small pieces before frying

Halloumi

Eggs:

Can be boiled or poached

The Simple Science Behind this Plan

The Ketogenic Diet or Keto is a low carbohydrate, high fat, moderate protein diet. On the Ketogenic Diet, your body enters a metabolic state called 'ketosis'. While in ketosis your body is using ketone bodies for energy instead of glucose. Ketone bodies are derived from fat and are a much more stable, steady source of energy than glucose, which is derived from carbohydrates.

This Ketogenic Plan promotes eating fresh, whole foods like meat, fish, vegetables and healthy fats and oils and eliminates the likes of processed and chemically treated foods. You can enter into a state of ketosis in as little as 24 hours using the recipes provided in this book. Once this occurs, you'll be using fat for energy, instead of carbohydrates.

This includes the fat you're eating from this high fat diet as well as your stored body fat. The meal plans I've created will help you to lose weight effortlessly while feeling satiated longer, thus helping to eliminate the desire to snack or overeat.

What is (IF)?

Intermittent Fasting or (IF) is currently one of the world's most popular health and fitness trends. People are using it to help them lose weight, improve their health and wellbeing and simplify their healthy lifestyles. Numerous studies show that it can have powerful effects on your body and brain and may even help you to live longer! Intermittent fasting (IF) is a term for an eating pattern that cycles between periods of fasting and eating. It doesn't focus on the foods you should eat, but rather when you should eat them. In this respect, it is not a "diet" in the conventional sense, it is more accurately described as an "eating pattern."Common intermittent fasting methods involve daily 16 hour fasts or fasting for 24 hours twice per week. I've chosen a daily 16 hour fast to include with this weight loss book as I've found it to be the easiest approach for me with my really hectic work life/family life schedule. As outlined in the 'Final Recap' section of the book - I chose to do the Intermittent Fasting between the hours of 8pm and 12pm daily. This meant that I was 'Fasting' overnight which made the plan much easier to maintain... at least initially until I entered 'ketosis'. Once I entered a state of ketosis I would find myself able to go much longer without meals as my body had begun burning my excess fat for energy!!

What to Be Aware Of?

Keto Flu is something that can happen when you suddenly remove or significantly reduce your intake of sugar/carbohydrates. Also known as the 'carb flu,' the keto flu is a natural reaction (almost like a feeling of withdrawal) your body undergoes when switching from burning glucose (sugar/carbohydrates) as energy to burning fat instead. Some common symptoms that can be experienced are: Fatigue, Headaches, Sniffles, Irritability & Nausea.

The main cause of keto flu is a sudden drop in sodium intake due to your eating habits changing to include more whole/natural foods while eliminating processed/chemically treated foods, so with that in mind, the keto flu can best be avoided by consuming enough electrolytes, especially sodium (hence the reason why Himalayan Sea Salt is included at almost every meal!)In addition, Himalayan Sea Salt can be sprinkled into drinking water and sipped on throughout the day if you are experiencing any of the symptoms above. Just be mindful that a little sprinkle is all that you need. Remember the saying **'LESS IS MORE'** and always opt for a high quality salt from your local health food store.

Final Recap

You will eat 3 meals per day for 7 days

Meals must be eaten within an 8 hour window i.e. between 12pm & 8pm (ideally you should eat at 12pm, 3pm and 7pm each day)

Meals cannot be changed around i.e. you can't eat breakfast from day 1 and the lunch from day 2 etc. However, if there is a particular day/days during the 7 day plan that you enjoy best then by all means repeat those days as often as you like over the 7 day period

You must drink 3 litres of water per day

You must drink 2 – 4 cups of caffeine free green tea each day

You may find the first couple of days a little difficult and you may experience some initial symptoms such as headache & low energy but worry not, this is just the body getting rid of excess insulin from your former carbohydrate-crazed diet!

When your body loses the initial weight, it can also lose electrolytes such as sodium, magnesium & potassium which is why you can often experience those symptoms.

Sipping on water that you've sprinkled with Himalayan sea salt can help to quickly replenish those electrolytes. So try it out... You'll be amazed to see how quickly those symptoms can disappear!

If you've enjoyed reading this book and have found my plan helpful please do be sure to rate and review it for me on Amazon. Thanks!

BONUS MATERIAL - 1 WEEK SHOPPING LIST & BEAUTIFULLY ILLUSTRATED RECIPE CHARTS THAT CAN BE PRINTED & LAMINATED & PLACED ON YOUR FRIDGE FOR A VISUAL GUIDE DURING THE 7 DAYS – Send me an Email to: nekinesiologist@hotmail.com requesting same. ☺

If you enjoyed my weight loss book – please do be sure to rate and review it for me on Amazon and keep an eye out for more low carbohydrate titles from me that are currently in the pipeline!

Other Notes:

If required you can choose the same quantity of fish for a meat dish or vice versa without it making too much of a difference or you can have chicken instead of turkey or vice versa.

To replace one egg in a recipe, whisk together 1 tablespoon of milled chia seeds or milled flaxseeds with 3 tablespoons of water until fully absorbed and thickened.

Future Plan:

This plan is very flexible and can be used in a number of ways:

Repeat the 1 week plan for up to 1 month or until you reach your goal weight.

Complete the 1 week plan then incorporate 2 days per week of the plan moving forward.

Complete the 1 week plan then continue to follow the plan every other day until your reach your goal weight.

Continue to incorporate the Intermittent Fasting 16:8 plan moving forward while choosing a number of meals from the 21 dishes provided to ensure you're keeping your carbohydrate/sugar intake low in order for you to maintain your goal weight.

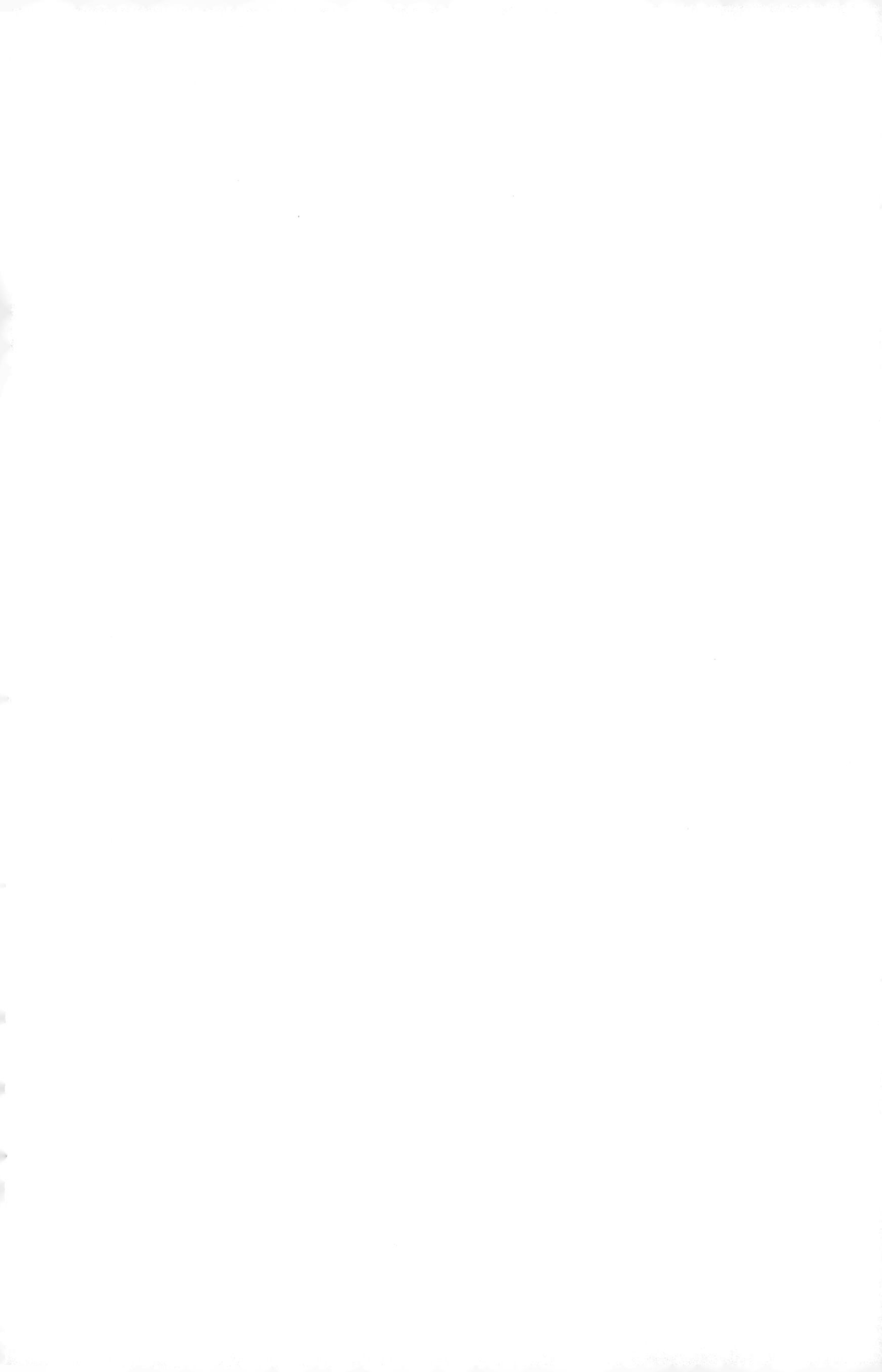

9 781659 493580